WALL PILATES FOR ELDERS

The Complete Guide to Reclaim Independence Mobility Balance, Fit and Posture with Simple 4-Week Whole Body Challenge Exercises.

RONALD P. SCOTT

DISCLAIMER

Please be aware that the material in this booklet is intended only for illustrative and recreational purposes. An enormous amount of work has gone into providing accurate, current, trustworthy, and comprehensive information. No express or implied guarantees of any sort are made. Readers understand that the author is not offering professional, legal, financial, or medical advice.

This book's material is a compilation of other sources. Please do not undertake any practices described in this book without first consulting a qualified specialist.

Upon perusing this document, the reader consents that the author will not be held accountable for any direct or indirect damages that may arise from utilizing the information provided herein, including but not limited to mistakes, omissions, or inaccuracies.

TABLE OF CONTENTS

"*Age is just a number, but strength is a choice.*"

INTRODUCTION

In his later years, Donald got renewed energy from the "Wall Pilate." He had battled with waning strength and flexibility at the age of 78. When he adopted this unusual workout routine, everything changed.

Donald would stand in front of the wall every morning, its surface changing into a painting of renewal. Pilate's Wall turned became his pillar of strength. He began with light stretches and worked his way up to more intense ones. His limbs were no longer rigid; they moved with elegance. With the wall as a constant, he was able to restore his equilibrium.

The regimen not only gave him his physical energy back, but it also lifted his spirits. He felt more energized and his posture straightened up, bringing him back to his younger self.

Donald defied his age and stood tall every day. He was able to enjoy the beauty of life's sunset with elegance and energy since The Wall Pilate was his hidden spring of youth.

Wall Pilates is a revolutionary workout program that shows you how to achieve long-term health and fitness.

In a world where the pressures of contemporary living often result in sedentary behaviors, Wall Pilates is a ray of light for those who want to be resilient and energetic. This unique combination of time-honored Pilates methods with the prop support of a wall may revitalize both the body and the mind.

The wall becomes a steady companion as one works with it, allowing for stretches, postures, and workouts that enhance balance, strength, and flexibility. Wall Pilates provides evidence that starting with a basic wall may lead to long-lasting fitness and energy on the path to maximum health.

WALL PILATES

Revolutionizing Health and Welfare

A unique combination of conventional Pilates methods and the use of a supported wall is known as wall Pilates. Utilizing the wall as a stabilizing assistance, this unique training routine applies the concepts of Pilates, stressing core strength, flexibility, balance, and the mind-body connection.

It is a flexible instrument that allows anyone, particularly seniors, to carry out a variety of exercises with additional assistance, guaranteeing both safety and efficient performance.

Wall Pilates' flexibility and accessibility are its main selling points. For a variety of stretches, postures, and motions, the wall provides stability and support. It provides a base for balance, enabling practitioners to experiment with a greater variety of exercises that may otherwise be difficult because of age-related restrictions or instability.

The emphasis on core strength in Wall Pilates is one of its main advantages. Practitioners build a stronger, more solid core by using the deep abdominal muscles, back muscles, and stabilizing muscles around the pelvis.

Better posture, less back discomfort, and improved general body control and alignment are the results of this.

Wall Pilates is also known for its flexibility. Stretching safely and effectively may be achieved by using the wall as a guide to increase flexibility in different muscle groups. People progressively extend their range of motion by doing mild stretches and wall exercises, which improves joint health and lowers the chance of injury.

Additionally, Wall Pilates improves stability and balance dramatically. Exercises that increase balance are especially beneficial for seniors since they reduce the risk of falls and boost self-assurance while doing regular tasks. Seniors may safely undertake balance-focused activities since the wall provides steady support.

It is impossible to ignore the mind-body connection that Wall Pilates promotes. It pushes practitioners to concentrate on deliberate movements and breathe work while being mindful of the current moment. This attentive method encourages mental clarity, stress reduction, and relaxation, all of which contribute to a comprehensive feeling of well-being.

The adaptability of Wall Pilates is one of its core principles. It may suit people with different degrees of ability and fitness. The wall offers a sturdy platform for the elderly or others with restricted mobility to execute activities that would otherwise appear difficult. On the other hand, expert practitioners might increase the level of difficulty or resistance in their exercises by adding a wall.

The variety of exercises offered by Wall Pilates is indicative of its versatility. Practitioners may customize their routines to match their unique requirements and objectives, ranging from mild stretches and strengthening exercises to dynamic postures and balancing problems. Wall Pilates provides a wide range of exercises that may be used to target certain muscle groups, increase flexibility, or concentrate on balance and coordination.

Furthermore, since Wall Pilates is a low-impact training technique that lessens joint stress and lowers the chance of injury, it is appropriate for people of all ages, especially seniors. Because of this, it's a great option for anybody searching for a safe and efficient way to maintain or increase their level of general fitness.

Wall Pilates has advantages that go beyond physical health. It encourages self-awareness and empowerment, boosting confidence and rekindling respect for the body's potential. Regular attendance at Wall Pilates may result in greater energy levels, better moods, and a feeling of achievement, all of which can enhance one's quality of life.

To put it simply, Wall Pilates is a comprehensive approach to health and fitness that provides a flexible and supportive framework for people, particularly seniors, to improve their core strength, flexibility, balance, and general vitality. It is a useful instrument for fostering mental clarity, physical health, and a fresh passion for life because of its accessibility, adaptability, and attentive practice.

50 WALL PILATES EXERCISES FOR ELDERS

The following list of 50 Wall Pilates exercises for elders includes suggested sets and repetitions along with introductions and instructions:

1. Hip Flexor Wall Stretch:

The goal of this exercise is to increase hip suppleness. With your back to the wall, plant one foot there and flex it gently.

Instructions: Bend forward and feel your hips expand. After twenty to thirty seconds of holding, swap legs.

Sets and Repetitions: Each leg receives two sets of three repetitions.

2. Wall Climbing:

Wall squats enhance balance and build stronger leg muscles. Place your feet shoulder-width apart and lean your back against the wall.

Instructions: Keep your back against the wall as you slowly lower yourself into a squat. Hold for a little while before getting back up.

Sets and Repetitions: Ten repetitions in two sets.

3. Panel Wall:

This workout improves stability and strength in the core. Assume a plank posture by facing the wall and resting your forearms against it.

Instruction: Maintain the plank posture for twenty to thirty seconds.

Sets and Repetitions: Three sets lasting twenty to thirty seconds each.

4. Wall Leg Lifts:

Take a position next to the wall and grasp it to develop your leg muscles.

Instruction: Raise one leg as high as comfortable and lower it down to the floor.

Sets and Repetitions: Each leg will do two sets of ten repetitions.

5. Wall push-ups:

Strengthen your upper body with wall push-ups. Stand with your arms outstretched, facing the wall.

Instructions: Push back to the starting position after lowering your chest toward the wall.

Sets & Repetitions: Ten repetitions in two sets.

6. Calf Raises on Walls:

The calf muscles are the focus of this workout. Place your hands on the wall for stability as you stand.

Instruction: Lift your heels to your toes and then drop them back down.

Sets and Repetitions: Three sets of fifteen reps each.

7. Wall Sit:

Wall sits improve the strength and stamina of the legs. Ascend to a sitting posture by leaning your back on the wall.

Instruction: Maintain the posture for the longest amount of time.

Sets And Repetitions: Two repetition in thirty second sets.

8. Wall-Made Chest Lock:

This exercise improves the flexibility of the chest and shoulders. Position yourself so that your hand is shoulder height away from the wall.

Instruction: Feel the strain in your chest as you slowly rotate your body away from the wall.

Sets and Repetitions: Twenty second sets on each side for two sets.

9. Stretch Your Wall Hamstrings:

This stretch increases the flexibility of the hamstrings. With your legs straight up the wall, lie on your back.

Instruction: Feel the stretch in your hamstrings as you gently push your heels on the wall.

Sets and Repetitions: Two thirty-second sets comprise the sets and repetitions.

10. Arm Circles on Walls:

Shoulder mobility may be improved by arm circles. Place your arms out in front of you as you face the wall.

Instruction: Move your arms in little circles and then in the other way.

Sets and Repetitions: 3 sets of 10 circles in each direction comprise the sets and repetitions.

11. Wall Leg Swings:

Wall leg swings increase hip flexion. Using one hand to steady yourself, stand close to the wall.

Instructions: Swing one leg straight forward and backward, then go on to the other leg.

Sets and Repetitions: Each leg will do two sets of fifteen swings.

12. Squeezing the wall shoulder blades:

Strengthen your upper back with this workout. Place your hands at chest height on the wall while standing facing it.

Instruction: Close your shoulders as if you're attempting to squeeze a pencil in between them.

Sets and Repetitions:: Three sets of fifteen squeezes each.

13. Dipping Wall Triceps:

The rear of the arms is the goal of tricep dips. Position your hands shoulder-width apart on the wall while standing with your back to it.

Instructions: Bend your elbows to lower your body, then push yourself back up.

Sets and Repetitions: Two sets of ten dips each.

14. Stretching the Wall Wrist Flexor:

Increase your wrist's flexibility with this stretch. Place your hand flat on the wall while facing it with your fingers pointed downward.

Instruction: Lean forward gently while noticing how your wrists are being stretched.

Sets and Repetitions: Each hand will do two sets of 20 seconds.

15. Knees to Chest on Wall:

This exercise increases the range of motion in the lower back and the hips. Place your buttocks against the wall while lying on your back.

Instructions: Feel a light lower back stretch as you hug your knees to your chest.

Sets & Repetitions: Ten repetitions in two sets.

16. Leg Raises along the Wall:

The outside thigh muscles are the focus of lateral leg lifts. For support, stand close to the wall.

Instruction: Raise one leg to the maximum comfortable height and then bring it back down.

Sets and Repetitions: Each leg will do two sets of ten lifts.

17. Glute Bridge Wall:

The lower back and glutes are strengthened via wall glute bridges. Lay flat on your back, knees bent, feet pressed up against the wall.

Instruction: Raise your hips off the floor, tighten your glutes, and then lower yourself back down.

Sets and Repetitions: Two pairs of fifteen bridges each.

18. Heel-to-toe Balance on the Wall:

This exercise improves ankle stability and balance. Grasp the wall with your fingers gently for stability as you stand.

Instruction: Step exactly in front of the other while walking in a straight line.

Sets and Repetitions: Two sets of ten steps each way comprise the sets and repetitions.

19. Twists of the wall abdomen:

The core muscles are worked during abdominal twists. With your back against the wall and your knees bent, take a seat on the floor.

Instruction: Rotate your body to twist to one side and then to the other.

Sets and Repetitions: There are three sets of fifteen twists each.

20. Wall Breathing:

This practice encourages mental clarity and relaxation. You may easily sit or stand with your back to the wall.

Instruction: Close your eyes, inhale deeply and slowly, and concentrate on the rise and fall of your belly and chest.

Sets and Repetitions: To lower stress and improve general well-being, practice for five to ten minutes each day.

21. Leg Raises from the Wall:

The hip and outer thigh muscles are worked during this workout. For support, stand with your side toward the wall.

Instruction: Raise one leg and then bring it back down.

Sets & Repetitions: Each leg will do twelve lifts in two sets.

22. Knee extensions with a wall seated:

The quadriceps are strengthened by this workout. With your feet flat on the wall, take a seat in a chair facing the wall.

Instruction: Lift your foot off the wall with one extended knee, then lower it.

Sets and Repetition: Each leg will do two sets of twelve extensions.

23. Wall Neck Extensions:

Neck stretches increase flexibility and reduce stress. Place your hand on the wall while standing with your side against it.

Instruction: Tilt your head gently to one side, maintain it there for 20 seconds, and then flip sides.

Sets and Repetitions: Twenty-second sets on each side for two sets.

24. Wall-side bends:

Increase your lateral flexibility with this workout. Place your side against the wall and your feet hip-width apart as you stand.

Instruction: Bend to the side and slide your hand down the wall, then come back up to a standing posture.

Sets & Repetition: Ten bends on each side in two sets.

25. Knee-to-Chest Stretch on the Wall:

This stretch enhances hip flexibility and releases tension in the lower back. Place your buttocks against the wall while lying on your back.

Instructions: Feel a little stretch in your lower back as you hug one knee to your chest.

Sets and Repetitions: Each leg should have two sets of ten stretches.

26. Extensor Wall Wrist Stretch:

This exercise improves the flexibility of the wrists. Place your hand flat on the wall while facing it with your fingers pointing upward.

Instructions: Feel the stretch in your wrist extensors as you gently lean forward.

Sets and Repetitions: Each hand will do two sets of twenty seconds.

27. Wall Knee Lifts:

The hip flexors are strengthened with knee raises. For support, stand close to the wall.

Instructions: Raise and then drop your knee to the level that feels comfortable.

Sets and Repetitions: Each leg receives two sets of ten lifts.

28. Retraction of the Wall Scapula:

Strengthen your upper back with this workout. Stand with your back to the wall and your arms outstretched to shoulder level.

Instructions: Squeeze and then release your shoulder blades.

Repetitions and Sets: Three sets of twelve retractions.

29. Alphabet on Wall Ankle:

Ankle mobility is enhanced with ankle alphabets. Place one foot against the wall while seated in a chair facing it.

Instructions: Move your ankle in different directions while using your toes to "write" the letters on the wall.

Sets and Repetition: Use each foot to finish the alphabet.

30. Quad Stretches on the Wall:

This stretch increases the flexibility of the quadriceps. Holding against the wall for support, stand facing it.

Instructions: Bend one knee and raise your heel to your buttocks while using your hand to grasp your foot.

Sets and Repetitions: Each leg will do two sets of fifteen seconds.

31. Hand Grips on Walls:

Strengthen your hands and forearms by using hand grips. With your back to the wall and your arms outstretched, take a stance facing it.

Instruction: Press your fingertips to the wall and then let go.

Repetitions and Sets: Three sets of twelve grips.

32. Wall Heel Lifts:

The calf muscles are the focus of heel raises. For support, place your fingers on the wall as you stand.

Instruction: Raise your heels to a comfortable level, then bring them back down.

Sets & Repetition: Two sets of fifteen lifts each.

33. Cat-Cow Wall Stretch:

This stretch releases stress from the back and increases spinal flexibility. Place your hands on the wall as you kneel in front of it.

Instructions: Push against the wall and arch your back (cow), then circle your back (cat).

Sets & Repetitions: Ten repetitions in two sets.

34. Circles of Wall Legs:

Hip mobility is enhanced by leg circles. Place one hand on the wall next to you for balance.

Instruction: Raise one leg and rotate it in both directions to create little circles.

Sets and Repetitions: Each leg will do two sets of ten circles.

35. Finger Taps on Walls:

Finger taps improve fine motor skills and hand-eye coordination. Assume a facing position and tap your fingers in different patterns on the wall.

Instruction: Tap your fingers in circles, up, down, left, and right.

Sets and Repetitions: Three sets of twenty taps each.

36. Pose of the Wall Child:

Lower back stretches and relaxation are enhanced by the child's position. With your arms outstretched and your forehead resting on the wall, kneel in front of it.

Instruction: Maintain the posture while concentrating on taking deep breaths and relaxing.

Sets and Repetitions: Two thirty-second sets comprise the sets and repetitions.

37. Curl Your Wall Biceps:

The arm muscles are the focus of bicep curls. Place your arms out in front of you as you face the wall.

Instructions: Curl your fists toward your shoulders by bending your elbows, then extend them.

Sets & Repetition: Twelve curls in two sets.

38. Hip Abduction Wall:

The outer hip muscles are strengthened via hip abduction. Holding onto the wall for support, stand with your side against it.

Instruction: Raise one leg and then bring it back down.

Sets and Repetitions: Each leg will do twelve lifts in two sets.

39. Twist Wall Standing:

Standing twists increase the flexibility of the spine. Place your arms out in front of you as you face the wall.

Instruction: Turn your body to one side while feeling the stretch in your back, then to the other.

Sets and Repetition: Each side does two sets of twelve twists.

40. Roll-down Walls:

This exercise improves the flexibility of the spine. Place your back against the wall and raise your arms over your head.

Instructions: Roll your spine slowly, one vertebra at a time, down toward the wall and back up.

Sets and Repetition: Roll downs in two sets of ten.

41. Extending the Wall Hip:

The lower back and glutes are strengthened via hip extensions. Place your hands on the wall for support as you stand facing it.

Instruction: Raise one leg straight behind you and then drop it back down.

Sets and Repetition: Each leg will do two sets of twelve extensions.

42. Knee Circles on Walls:

Knee circles improve the flexibility and range of motion in the hips. Place one hand on the wall next to you for balance.

Instruction: Raise your knee and rotate in a circle, going in one way at first and then the other.

Sets and Repetitions: Each leg will do two sets of ten circles.

43. Shoulder blade squeezes with the wall reversed:

Squeezing your shoulders backward may help with posture and upper back strength. Stand with your back to the wall and your arms outstretched to shoulder level.

Instruction: Squeeze your shoulder blades together and push your chest forward, then let go.

Sets and Repetitions: Three sets of twelve squeezes each.

44. Hamstring Curl on Wall:

The back of the thighs are strengthened with hamstring curls. Holding the wall for support, stand facing it.

Instructions: Extend your leg back after bending one knee and pulling your heel near your buttocks.

Sets and Repetitions: Each leg will do two sets of ten curls.

45. Circles of Wall Foot:

Ankle circulation and mobility are enhanced by foot circles. Place one foot up against the wall while seated in a chair facing it.

Instruction: Make circular movements with your ankle, rotating it first in one way and then the other.

Sets and Repetition: Each foot will do two sets of ten circles.

46. Quad Stretch on Wall:

Stretching the quadriceps increases their flexibility. Holding against the wall for support, stand facing it.

Instructions: Bend one knee and raise your heel to your buttocks while using your hand to grasp your foot.

Sets and Repetitions: Each leg will do two sets of fifteen seconds.

47. Wall Arm Swings:

Shoulder mobility is enhanced by arm swings. Place your arms out in front of you as you face the wall.

Instruction: Make controlled movements with your arms as you swing them forth and backward.

Repetitions and Sets: Three sets of ten swings each.

48. Hip Circles on Walls:

Hip circles increase the flexibility and mobility of the hips. You can place one of your hands on the next wall to you for support.

Instruction: Move your hips in a circle, starting in one direction and working your way to the other.

Sets and Repetitions: Two sets of ten circles in each direction comprise the sets and repetitions.

49. Taps on Wall Legs:

Leg taps improve balance and leg strength. Place one hand on the wall for support as you stand facing it.

Instruction: Raise one leg, tap it out to the side, and then lower it back to the center.

Sets and Repetition: Each leg receives two sets of twelve taps.

50. Wall Bridge:

The lower back, hamstrings, and glutes are strengthened via wall bridges. Lay flat on your back with your legs bent and your feet flat on the wall.

Instruction: Raise your hips off the floor, tighten your glutes, and then lower yourself back down.

Sets and Repetitions: Two sets of twelve.

MOTIVATIONAL QUOTES

The following 20 quotes might be appropriate for you in the journey of "Wall Pilates".

These quotations might act as energizing prompts to encourage and inspire you to start Wall Pilates.

1. *"Feeling flexible, strong, and full of life is never too late.*

2. *"Age is just a number, but strength is a choice."*

3. *"With the wall as your support, every challenge becomes an opportunity for growth."*

4. *"Instead of just using the wall as a dramatic prop, Wall Pilate utilizes it as a symbol of power."*

5. *"Embrace the wisdom of your years and the power of Wall Pilates to create a life of vitality."*

6. *"The body's potential knows no age limit."*

7. *"Strength doesn't come from what you can do; it comes from overcoming the things you once thought you couldn't."*

8. *"The wall is your ally on the path to a healthier, more vibrant you."*

9. *"With each Wall Pilates session, you're writing your own story of resilience and transformation."*

10. *"Giving your body Pilates is a gift." Welcome it, hold it close, and allow it to uplift your soul."*

11. *"Being older is a chance. The vehicle is Pilates."*

12. *"Wall Pilates: Where decision meets the wall, and strength flourishing."*

13. *The most valuable thing you own is your body. Wall Pilates may help you take care of it."*

14. *"Your being exceptional than what you were yesterday is what matters, not being the finest*

15. *"As your body processes everything that you are thinking, give it courage and positivity."*

16. *"The journey to health and vitality begins one Wall Pilates session at a time."*

17. *"With every wall-supported stretch, you're reaching for a better version of yourself."*

18. *"More significant than the amount of days you have lived on Earth is your year of healthy living. Wall Pilates assists you in making the most of each year.*

19. *"Your attitude decides your ability; not your age. Use Wall Pilates to empower yourself.*

20. *"Wall Pilate is irreplaceable as the only means of ultimate testimonial."*

CONCLUSION

Towards the end of "Wall Pilates for Elders," you should take a moment to consider the amazing trip you have already on. For seniors, this book has been a key to a happier, healthier, and more satisfying existence where becoming older doesn't mean losing vitality—rather, it's a springboard to newfound energy.

As we get to the end of our trip, keep in mind that the wall has served as a metaphor of your steadfast fortitude and perseverance in addition to providing physical support. It has seen your growth, your will to conquer obstacles, and your dedication to improving your wellbeing.

You've learned that every day is a chance to improve your strength, flexibility, and awareness of your body thanks to Wall Pilates. You've accepted the advice of experience and used Pilates to enhance your physical and mental health.

I hope this book serves as a reminder that you may always choose to live your best life and that age is only a number. Your experience with Wall Pilates is evidence of your resilient nature and limitless potential.

Allow it to serve as a source of encouragement and inspiration for you to keep moving in the direction of a life that is full of elegance, health, and energy. We are grateful that Wall Pilates could be a part of your incredible experience.